ATOPIC DERMATITIS

Comprehensive Strategies for Clear and Healthy Skin: The Atopic Dermatitis Handbook

CARL JUAN

Table of Contents

Introductory

Common and persistent, atopic dermatitis (or "eczema") is characterized by skin inflammation and irritation. Rashes appear on the skin and can itch, dry, turn red, and even ooze. Dermatitis, which includes atopic dermatitis, refers to inflammation of the skin.

Certain characteristics of atopic dermatitis are:

- One of the most noticeable symptoms is itching. Scratching, which can make the itching worse, can be a vicious cycle.

• Inflammation and redness can appear on the skin in affected areas.

• Dry skin is characterized by a lack of moisture, which causes it to become rough and scaly.

• Eczema rashes are characterized by itchy, red areas of skin that may bleed and harden over time.

• It can show up anywhere on the body, but usually it's in creases of skin, like the creases inside the elbows or the creases at the back of the knees. In babies, it can affect the face, scalp, and other places.

Flare-ups and remissions are both possible with a chronic illness like atopic dermatitis. It usually manifests itself in early childhood, but it's possible for it to develop or continue into maturity. Although the precise causes of atopic dermatitis are unknown, it is thought that genetic, environmental, and immune system variables all play a role.

Common practices for treating atopic dermatitis include:

• Moisturizers, corticosteroid creams, and non-steroidal anti-inflammatory creams are examples of topical treatments that can be applied directly to the skin to alleviate redness, swelling, and itching.

• Recognizing and avoiding the soaps, detergents, or allergies that aggravate your condition is an important part of managing your symptoms.

• Modifications to Your Way of Life: Drinking enough of water and avoiding long, hot showers are only two examples.

• Oral medicines or immunosuppressant may be prescribed by a doctor in extreme situations.

- In circumstances where allergies are a contributing factor, allergen testing may be required for diagnosis and management of the condition.

It's crucial for persons with atopic dermatitis to engage closely with a healthcare provider to build a specific treatment plan to manage their condition properly. Although a solution has not been discovered for atopic dermatitis, the condition can be managed to alleviate symptoms and enhance quality of life.

CHAPTER ONE
Impact and Prevalence

Atopic dermatitis (eczema) is quite common and can have serious consequences that change with age, location, and the individual. Take a look at this synopsis of its widespread effects:

Prevalence:

• Atopic dermatitis is one of the most prevalent skin conditions worldwide. Although it can start at any age, early childhood is a common onset time.

• Beginning in childhood, up to 20% of children in developed countries will acquire eczema at some point in their lives. Many of these kids grow out of it or have less severe symptoms as they get older.

• Both the persistence of and the onset of atopic dermatitis in adulthood are possible. Although less common in adults, the condition can still cause serious problems.

• The incidence of atopic dermatitis varies from one geographic area and demographic to another. It occurs more frequently in industrialized nations, especially in metropolitan areas.

Impact:

• **Quality of Life:** Atopic dermatitis can have a profound impact on a person's quality of life. Skin rashes can cause severe physical and mental anguish due to their acute itching, discomfort, and appearance.

• Psychological Impact The outward manifestation of this disorder can cause its sufferers, particularly teenagers and adults, to experience feelings of shame and low self-esteem. It could cause emotional and interpersonal issues in the long run.

- In extreme cases, atopic dermatitis can cause disruptions in daily life, including trouble sleeping and difficulty concentrating in the classroom.

- Scratching because you're itchy increases your risk of developing a skin infection, scars, or even a change in skin tone. This can further increase the impact of the illness.

- The financial impact of managing atopic dermatitis can be significant due to the potential need for expensive treatment options such as prescription drugs, office visits, and over-the-counter products.

- Atopic dermatitis is one of the three conditions that make up the atopic triad, the other two being asthma and allergic rhinitis (hay fever). This suggests that those with eczema may also be more susceptible to these diseases.

- Atopic dermatitis is a chronic illness characterized by remission and flare-up. This ongoing nature of the problem may exacerbate its long-term effects on affected people and their loved ones.

Atopic dermatitis is a major public health problem because of its high incidence and potential for serious personal and family consequences.

Minimizing its effects and improving the quality of life for people who are afflicted requires proper care, which includes early diagnosis and adequate therapy. Atopic dermatitis management can also entail providing information and resources to patients and their loved ones so they can better manage the condition.

Factors That Set It Off

Atopic dermatitis (eczema) is thought to be caused by a mix of genetic, environmental, and immune system factors, although the specific causes are not known. The illness might manifest differently in different people, and its source is unknown. Some of the following are hypothesized to play a role in the onset or worsening of atopic dermatitis:

1. In terms of genetics, it's important to consider your family history. If one or both parents have a history of atopic dermatitis, asthma, or allergic rhinitis, a child is at a higher risk of acquiring eczema.

2. An overreaction of the immune system is linked to atopic dermatitis. Inflammation and other skin signs may result from an immune system's overreaction to several causes.

3. Atopic dermatitis sufferers frequently have a compromised skin barrier. Causes inflammation and other symptoms by facilitating the entry of irritants, allergens, and germs into the skin.

4. Pollen, animal dander, dust mites, and mold are just some of the environmental allergens that have been linked to eczema flare-ups.

5. Causes of eczema flare-ups include contact with irritants such as harsh soaps, detergents, and some skin care products.

6. Weather and climate can play a role in exacerbating eczema symptoms, since dry air, low humidity, and freezing temperatures can all aggravate the condition.

7. Some people, especially youngsters, are predisposed to developing eczema due to allergies to certain foods or other chemicals.

8. Some people's eczema's occurrence and severity can be affected by hormonal shifts that occur throughout puberty, pregnancy, and menopause.

9. Emotional and mental stressors have been linked to exacerbation of eczema symptoms. The use of

stress-reduction strategies may aid in the treatment of the illness.

10. Infections such as bacteria, viruses, or fungi can aggravate eczema. Scratching can also cause infections because it opens the skin to microorganisms.

11. The symptoms of eczema can be triggered or made worse by food allergies, especially in newborns and young children. Dairy, eggs, nuts, and shellfish are common allergens.

Identifying and avoiding certain triggers is an important aspect of controlling atopic dermatitis. It's important to remember that each person's eczema is unique, and what aggravates one person's condition may have no effect on another. Individuals with eczema may benefit from working closely with healthcare providers to identify personal triggers and create a tailored management strategy. To manage symptoms and forestall flare-ups, this strategy may involve modifying one's way of life, instituting skin care routines, and, in some situations, taking medication.

CHAPTER TWO
Symptoms and Indicators

The signs and symptoms of atopic dermatitis (eczema) vary from person to person, as does the disease's severity. Atopic dermatitis typically manifests with the following signs and symptoms:

• One of the most noticeable and bothersome symptoms of eczema is pruritus, or itching. Scratching, in response to the extreme itching, might make the problem worse.

• **Red or Inflamed Skin:** Affected parts of the skin often become red and inflamed. The level of redness, if any, may change.

- **Rough, Scaly, or Cracked Skin:** Eczema-prone skin tends to be dry and flaky.

- Red pimples, blisters, or papules could appear on your skin if you have eczema. These may develop a crusty ooze over time.

- Edema, or localized swelling, is a common symptom of eczema.

- Vesicles, or blisters, are tiny, fluid-filled bumps that might appear on afflicted areas in certain people.

- **Thickened Skin:** Over time, the skin in chronic eczema instances can become thickened and leathery, a condition known as lichenification.

- Excessive moisture: eczema, especially in newborns, can cause the skin to become weepy or ooze.

- **Skin Sensitivity:** Eczema-prone skin is particularly vulnerable to irritants like harsh soaps and detergents, which can cause an immediate reaction.

- Open sores caused by scratching sensitive skin are a breeding ground for bacteria and fungi, making the affected areas more susceptible to infection.

- Eczema rashes can appear in different places at different ages. In infants, it is usually present on the face, scalp, and trunk. It can appear anywhere on the body, but is most common in skin folds like the insides of the elbows and the backs of the knees in both children and adults.

- The chronic, relapsing-remitting nature of eczema means that symptoms may subside for a period before flaring up again.

The degree and presentation of symptoms might vary considerably between individuals. Some people only have minor, intermittent symptoms, while others have severe, chronic eczema. Controlling symptoms and increasing quality of life for persons with atopic dermatitis require proper management and treatment, which may include moisturizers, topical corticosteroids, and other drugs. Also important in controlling this disease is learning to recognize and avoid triggers. If you or a loved one is having symptoms consistent with atopic dermatitis, it is best to get a proper diagnosis and treatment from a medical practitioner.

Assessing and Diagnosing

Atopic dermatitis (eczema) is diagnosed and evaluated using a mix of clinical examination, patient history, and occasionally, further diagnostic procedures. The procedure usually goes like this:

1. A doctor, typically a dermatologist, will perform a physical examination of the affected areas of skin. Redness, dryness, rashes, and itching are all symptoms commonly associated with eczema, thus these will all be checked for. The geographic dispersion of these signs is also documented.

The provider may inquire as to the rash's location and how it looks to have a better idea of what's going on.

2. Health Background:

• Since atopic dermatitis frequently includes a hereditary component, it is important to know whether or not the patient has a personal and/or family history of eczema or other allergic illnesses.

• Exposure to allergens or irritants, for example, may be brought up as a possible trigger and aggravating factor, and the patient's history of these may be examined.

Asking the patient about their lifestyle, including their diet, exercise routine, and usage of skincare products, can provide insight into possible underlying factors.

3. Evaluations and Checkups:

• It may be necessary to perform a skin prick test to determine whether allergens are causing or exacerbating the eczema in a given individual. This entails putting a tiny amount of an allergen to the skin and testing for a reaction.

• Allergens and foods that trigger them can be pinpointed with the use of blood tests like the specialized IgE tests.

The use of a skin biopsy to rule out other skin disorders that can mimic eczema is reserved for extremely unusual circumstances.

4. Rating the Degree of Illness:

• Tools like these are commonly used to evaluate the severity of atopic dermatitis:

• A scoring method that takes into account both the afflicted area and the intensity of symptoms including redness, itching, and swelling is the Eczema Area and Severity Index (EASI).

• Scoring Atopic Dermatitis (SCORAD): SCORAD is another instrument used to measure the extent and severity of eczema, taking into account various symptoms and their impact on the patient's quality of life.

• Patient-Reported Outcomes: Itchiness, sleep disturbances, and quality of life are all things that patients can report on to assist doctors gauge the severity of eczema's effects.

5. Diagnostic Variation:

• When diagnosing eczema, doctors must first rule out less common causes of the skin rash, such as contact dermatitis, psoriasis, seborrheic dermatitis, and fungal infections.

• After a diagnosis has been made, the doctor will work with the patient to develop a treatment plan that may include dietary and lifestyle changes, advice on skin care, and possibly pharmaceuticals like topical corticosteroids, calcineurin inhibitors, or antihistamines. The purpose of treatment is to alleviate suffering by controlling symptoms and avoiding exacerbations.

A chronic condition with varied triggers and treatment responses, atopic dermatitis generally requires continuing assessment and follow-up with a healthcare provider to ensure the best effective management approach for each individual.

CHAPTER THREE
Alternative Treatments

Symptom relief, reduced inflammation, prevention of flare-ups, and an enhanced quality of life are common goals of treatment for those who suffer with atopic dermatitis (eczema). Atopic dermatitis treatments may include:

• Regular use of emollients (moisturizers) is essential for eczema therapy. These creams help hydrate and protect the skin, minimizing dryness and irritation. Thick emollients like creams and ointments are commonly suggested.

- Anti-inflammatory creams or ointments, known as topical corticosteroids, are widely administered for eczema patients to alleviate symptoms of inflammation and itching. The options range from moderate to vigorous, with the milder ones being used on the face and genitalia.

- Topical calcineurin inhibitors, such tacrolimus (Protopic) and pimecrolimus (Elidel), are non-steroidal topical drugs that can relieve inflammation and itching, even in delicate areas like the face, neck, and skin folds.

• Crisaborole (Eucrisa), a member of the non-steroidal topical drug class known as phosphodiesterase-4 inhibitors, is used to treat mild to moderate cases of atopic dermatitis in both children and adults.

• Creams developed to help restore the skin's natural barrier, which is frequently damaged by eczema, are available for topical use. They have the potential to boost skin health and minimize moisture loss.

• Antihistamines, either over-the-counter or prescribed, can help with itching and discomfort, especially if it's keeping you up at night.

• After medication has been applied to the skin, wet wrap therapy entails wrapping the area in a moist bandage or dressing to increase moisture and reduce inflammation.

• Treatment of severe eczema that hasn't improved with other methods may include exposure to ultraviolet (UV) light in a medical setting. This is something that is usually done in a clinical context.

• In extreme cases, or when other therapies have failed, systemic drugs such as oral corticosteroids or immunosuppressant's such as cyclosporine or methotrexate may be used. Due to the higher risk of adverse effects, these drugs are only ever taken under strict medical care.

• Some people who have specific allergies that cause eczema have found relief with allergen immunotherapy (such as allergy injections) to be helpful.

• Modifying one's way of life and taking precautions at home can be equally important in the treatment and management of eczema as conventional medical methods. Cases in point may include:

• Recognizing and avoiding allergies and irritants.

Taking brief, lukewarm showers and avoiding vigorous scrubbing are all part of good skin care practices.

You can help by dressing in breathable, soft fabrics.

- Managing stress: Stress management practices can help prevent flare-ups.

It's crucial for persons with eczema to engage closely with a healthcare professional to build a specific treatment strategy. Symptom management and flare-up avoidance are best achieved with a multipronged strategy.

Additionally, individuals and their families should receive knowledge and support to effectively manage eczema and improve their quality of life.

Managing Atopic Dermatitis in Daily Life

Atopic dermatitis (eczema) can be difficult to live with, but there are many things one can do to better control their symptoms and enhance their quality of life. Suffering with atopic dermatitis? Here are some pointers:

1. Create Your Own Skincare Regimen:

• Keep your skin nourished by using mild cleansers and fragrance-free moisturizers.

• Moisturize right after a shower to prevent water loss.

Showers and baths should be kept short and lukewarm rather than hot.

• Use a soft towel to pat dry the skin instead of rubbing.

2. Recognize and Sidestep Triggers:

• Discuss potential eczema aggravating factors with your doctor.

• Stay away from soaps, detergents, and materials that are known to aggravate or trigger allergies.

• Alter your routine to reduce the number of times you're exposed to triggers.

3. Dress appropriately:

• Fabrics that are rough or scratchy should be avoided in favor of softer, more breathable ones such as cotton.

Layer your clothing so you may easily alter it for warmth or coolness.

4. Stress Management:

• Stress can make eczema worse. Take some deep breaths, meditate, or do some yoga to calm your nerves.

If stress becomes overwhelming, it may be time to consult a mental health expert.

5. Eat Consciously:

• See an allergist for testing if you believe food allergies are the cause of your eczema.

• Do what your doctor says in terms of your diet.

6. Avoid dehydration:

• Drinking enough water will help keep your skin hydrated from the inside out.

7. Take Prescription Drugs as Directed:

• If your doctor recommends a topical cream or an oral treatment, use it as instructed.

8. How to Stop Scratching:

• Keep your nails short to reduce skin injury from scratching.

To relieve itching, try using cool compresses.

• Take antihistamines, either over-the-counter or prescribed by your doctor.

9. Get the facts and get some help:

• Get informed from reliable sources on atopic dermatitis and its treatment.

Connect with individuals who understand what it's like to live with eczema by joining a support group or an online community.

10. Maintaining Frequent Contact with Your Healthcare Provider:

• In order to monitor your progress and make any necessary adjustments to your treatment plan, it is important to schedule follow-up consultations with your doctor on a frequent basis.

11. Record Your Symptoms:

• If you want to figure out what's causing your symptoms, it can help to keep track of when and where they occur, as well as any changes to your routine.

12. Maintain Your Knowledge on Recent Medical Developments

• New methods of therapy and care are being developed all the time. Get the latest information about treatment choices from doctors and medical groups.

Remember that atopic dermatitis is a chronic illness that might vary in its course from person to person. There may not be a cure, but your symptoms can be greatly diminished with the help of treatment, and your overall quality of life can increase. Don't give up hope, and don't be shy about consulting with medical experts for advice on how to best manage your illness.

CHAPTER FOUR
Maintenance and Safety Measures

Preventing and effectively managing atopic dermatitis (eczema) frequently involves a combination of strategies to lessen the frequency and severity of flare-ups. Long-term management of eczema attempts to offer relief and improve quality of life despite the lack of a cure. Some methods of avoidance and long-term control are as follows:

1. Maintenance of the Skin:

- Use a moisturizer on a regular basis to maintain your skin supple and nourished. Moisturize using hypoallergenic, fragrance-free products.

• When bathing, use soft, non-soap cleansers and take brief, lukewarm baths or showers. Avoid hard scrubbing, which can further irritate the skin.

Applying a moisturizer right after a shower is the quickest way to lock in moisture.

• Stay away from irritants by only using fragrance-free, gentle cleaning and personal care items. Eczema flare-ups can be prevented by avoiding items with strong chemicals and smells.

2. Recognize and Sidestep Triggers:

• Consult with a doctor or allergist to narrow down the list of potential allergens and irritants that set off your eczema. Take steps to avoid or reduce exposure to these triggers.

3. Changes in How You Live:

• If your eczema flares up after eating particular foods, talk to your doctor about making dietary adjustments.

• Stress Management: Practice relaxation methods like deep breathing, meditation, or yoga to alleviate the effects of stress on your skin, which can make eczema worse.

4. Medications:

• In the event of an outbreak, it is recommended that you use any topical drugs (such as corticosteroids or calcineurin inhibitors) prescribed by your doctor.

Your doctor may recommend oral drugs for more severe cases, but you should use them with caution and under medical supervision due to the risk of adverse consequences.

5. Phototherapy:

• Phototherapy (Light Therapy): If your severe eczema isn't responding to other treatments, talk to your doctor about trying phototherapy (light therapy).

6. Immunotherapy with Allergens:

• Allergen immunotherapy (allergy shots): If allergies are a recognized trigger for your eczema, this treatment may help alleviate your symptoms.

7. Ongoing Monitoring:

• Healthcare Provider Visits: Schedule regular follow-up appointments with your healthcare provider to check your condition and make necessary adjustments to your treatment plan.

8. Instruction and Assistance:

• Get informed. Read more about eczema and how to treat it at credible websites. As a result, you'll have a greater grasp of the situation and be more equipped to make wise choices.

Join a local eczema support group or an online community where you can talk to people who understand what you're going through. It's helpful to share stories and tips.

9. Record Your Symptoms:

• Keep a diary of your symptoms, any changes to your routine or exposure to probable triggers, and the times and places that you experience flare-ups. This might be useful for spotting trends.

10. Prolonged Dedication:

• Consistency: Realize that long-term eczema control calls for steady work. It may take some time before you see any changes, and you may still get flare-ups.

Always keep in mind that finding an approach that works for your atopic dermatitis is a continuous journey. Creating a tailor-made management strategy requires close collaboration with your healthcare provider. Although atopic dermatitis can be difficult to control, doing so over time can greatly lessen symptoms and boost quality of life.

Conclusion

Atopic dermatitis, often known as eczema, is a chronic skin disorder that affects a large percentage of the general population. Although eczema has no known treatment, it can be controlled and lived with using a variety of methods. Preventative measures, therapeutic measures, and ongoing administration are all included.

• Prevention entails identifying and avoiding triggers, controlling stress, and implementing a mild skincare routine. The key to reducing flare-ups is pinpointing the exact allergens or irritants that trigger them. Modifications to one's way of life, such as those involving one's nutrition and stress management practices, can also play an important part in the avoidance of eczema.

• Depending on the severity of the problem, treatment options range from using moisturizers and topical drugs to using oral meds and phototherapy. These remedies are meant to ease discomfort, calm inflammation, and enhance skin health.

• Consistent and patient effort is required for long-term management of eczema. Effective eczema management requires a number of steps, including regular follow-up with healthcare experts, knowledge about the illness, and finding support from those who have gone through something similar.

Although atopic dermatitis can make day-to-day life difficult, it is possible to live a full and productive life with the correct approach and assistance. Patients with eczema should collaborate closely with their doctors to create a treatment plan that is tailored to their specific condition and symptoms.

THE END

www.ingramcontent.com/pod-product-compliance
Lightning Source LLC
Chambersburg PA
CBHW071019260726
48662CB00022B/780